# MULTIPLE CHOICE QUESTIONS ON
# LECTURE NOTES ON
# GENERAL SURGERY

# Multiple Choice Questions on Lecture Notes on General Surgery

**P. R. FLEMING,** MD FRCP
Senior Lecturer in Medicine
Charing Cross and Westminster Medical School

**J. F. STOKES,** MD FRCP
Formerly Consultant Physician
University College Hospital, London

**T. COOKE,** MD FRCS
Senior Lecturer in Surgery
University of Liverpool

*Foreword by*
HAROLD ELLIS, MA MCh DM FRCS
Professor of Surgery
Charing Cross and Westminster Medical School

*THIRD EDITION*

BLACKWELL SCIENTIFIC PUBLICATIONS
OXFORD LONDON EDINBURGH
BOSTON PALO ALTO MELBOURNE

First published 1977
Second edition 1980
Third edition 1987

Set by Katerprint Typesetting
Services, Oxford, England
Printed in Great Britain by
Billing & Sons Ltd, Worcester

DISTRIBUTORS

USA
  Year Book Medical Publishers
  35 East Wacker Drive
  Chicago, Illinois 60601

Canada
  The C. V. Mosby Company
  5240 Finch Avenue East
  Scarborough, Ontario

Australia
  Blackwell Scientific Publications
    (Australia) Pty Ltd
  107 Barry Street
  Carlton, Victoria 3053

British Library
Cataloguing in Publication Data

Fleming, P. R.
  Multiple choice questions on
  Lecture notes on general
  surgery. — 3rd ed.
  1. Surgery — Problems,
  exercises, etc.
  I. Title   II. Stokes, J. F.
  III. Cooke, T.
  IV. Ellis, Harold, *1926*– Lecture
  notes on general surgery
  617′.0076    RD37.2

  ISBN 0-632-01664-7

# CONTENTS

FOREWORD *by Professor Harold Ellis*     vii

HOW TO USE THIS BOOK     1

PART ONE     5
*Independent True/False*
*by chapter*

PART TWO     48
Section A: *Independent True/False*     48
Section B: *One-from-Five*     57
Section C: *Relationship Analysis*     61

ANSWERS
*Part One*     64
*Part Two*     66

# FOREWORD

The MCQ has come to stay in the examination system of this and many other countries. Of course it has its disadvantages—it is impersonal, it does not test the candidate's ability to express himself in English or to display his processes of logical thought (but other parts of the examination can do this) and it lacks fine gradations of meaning. Yet, it does enable a wide field of factual knowledge to be tested and no-one can accuse the computer of marking unfairly. It also serves another useful purpose in that it enables the student to check his knowledge-store and to ensure that he has absorbed at least the essentials of any programme of study.

I have had an enjoyable experience working through this volume. If it is of any satisfaction to the reader, I confess that I made some mistakes, although I do not think these were very serious ones. At the request of the authors I have indicated, by asterisks against the question numbers in the Answers section, those which seem to me to deal with the most important aspects of general surgery. Errors in these questions suggest that careful re-reading of the topic is required; these are subjects which most examiners would expect the student to be quite clear in his mind about and in which muddled thinking and ignorance might lead to some unpleasant disasters in an oral examination.

Dr Peter Fleming, Dr John Stokes and Mr Timothy Cooke, three seasoned experts in the construction of MCQ, have provided what I believe is a most useful set of questions for the student, as well as a helpful introductory guide to answering them. The need for a third edition is sufficient proof of the continued value and popularity of this book.

*Harold Ellis*

# HOW TO USE THIS BOOK

It will not have escaped the notice of most medical students that multiple choice questions (MCQ) are playing an increasingly large part in the various examinations which punctuate the undergraduate medical course. MCQ are admittedly not universally popular, especially among examination candidates, but most examiners find them far too useful to consider abandoning this technique and it must be assumed that MCQ have come to stay in one form or another.

Apart from their use in formal examinations, assessment techniques, including MCQ, have an important part to play in the educational process itself. Unless you are blessed with a phenomenal memory, it is wise to pause frequently while studying to ask yourself whether you have remembered and understood what you have just been learning. This informal self-assessment can, we believe, be made more searching and, therefore, more useful by the use of questions based on the material which has been studied. MCQ are particularly useful in this respect and it is mainly with this purpose in mind that this book has been written. In this third edition we have updated Parts 1 and 2 to keep abreast of changes in surgical management and added further questions to Part 2.

## MCQ AS A METHOD OF CONTINUOUS SELF-ASSESSMENT

The questions in Part 1 of this book are arranged according to the chapters in *Lecture Notes on General Surgery* on which they are based. This section has been revised to correspond with the sixth edition of Lecture Notes. We suggest that, after you have read a few pages or a chapter or two, you attempt to answer the appropriate questions and check your accuracy against the Answer Key at the back of this book. In most cases, the Answer Key simply lists the correct items in each question but occasionally when, in the view of the authors of the Lecture Notes, a wrong answer indicates a serious, or dangerous, lack of knowledge, an asterisk is appended. In any case you are strongly advised to refer to the original text whenever you have incorrectly identified an item as *True* or *False* to see how your error has arisen. You should not expect to be able to answer all the MCQ correctly at a first reading; indeed, if you *are* able to do so, you should probably be reading a larger textbook on the subject or, better, applying your knowledge in the wards. Another important point is that it is not possible to test your knowledge of all the information contained in the Lecture Notes by means of MCQ and you should not assume that, because you can answer the questions correctly, you are fully conversant with the subject. Answering the MCQ will give you a very fair idea of the extent of your factual knowledge but will rarely allow you to assess your ability to marshal facts and to reason logically about them. You should, therefore, continue to check your skill in this area by other means, such as discussion with your colleagues and your teachers.

All the MCQ in Part 1 of this book are of the *Independent True/False* type, that is in any question any number of items, or all or none of them, may be correct. Questions in other formats appear in Part 2 which is discussed below.

## MCQ IN EXAMINATIONS

In Part 2 which has been extended for this edition the MCQ are not arranged in parallel with the chapters of the corresponding Lecture Notes although all of them deal with material which can be found there. They can be used, therefore, for revision when the whole of the book has been read or, independently of the Lecture Notes, as part of your preparation for a formal examination in which MCQ are used. The questions in Part 1 can, of course, also be used for this purpose. In Part 2 apart from the questions in the *Independent True/False* format (Section A), some are of the *One-from-Five* type which is used in some examinations (Section B). In the latter, *only one* of the items is correct and, if you should meet questions of this type, it is clearly important not to confuse them with those in the *Independent True/False* format. There will usually be clear instructions on the examination paper to prevent this confusion. Another type of question which is used in Part 2 is the *Relationship Analysis* in which you are given two statements linked by the word 'because' (Section C). You have to decide whether one or both statements are true and, if both are true, whether the second is a correct explanation of the first; further details are given in Part 2.

A final few words of advice on the tactics to be adopted when answering MCQ in examinations may be helpful. It goes without saying that the best way to do well in a MCQ paper is to be thoroughly well-informed about the subject. However, few are without gaps, of varying size, in their knowledge and it is sensible to give some thought to how best to use such knowledge as you possess. You will usually find that you are asked to indicate, for each item in each question, whether you regard it as True or False; in most examinations, you have a third option — that of omitting the item altogether. If this is the case, you will be faced with the problem of how much to 'guess'.

Temperaments differ and each of you will have a, more or less strong, natural inclination to guess or not to guess. Before allowing your natural inclinations full play, however, it is wise to consider the problem rationally. There will, we hope, be some items about which you are in no doubt and you can clearly answer them confidently as True or False. There will, probably, be other items about which you are totally ignorant. With most of the marking systems in use, in which marks are deducted for wrong answers, there is nothing to be gained by guessing the answers to such items and you should omit them.

The most important items, from the point of view of doing yourself justice, are those about which you are not quite certain and yet they 'ring a bell'. Even if your knowledge of the subject is somewhat hazy, it is likely that you will have a 'hunch' about the right answer and as, on balance, hunches are more often correct than not, you should answer such questions accordingly. This is not really 'guessing' but rather taking action on the basis of incomplete knowledge. Such action would not be regarded as reprehensible in a clinician who is forced by the severity of his patient's illness to begin treatment before he is completely certain of the diagnosis. It is no more reprehensible in an examination candidate and is, usually, profitable when he is faced by MCQ of this nature.

# PART ONE

In this part all of the questions are of the *Independent True/ False* type, i.e. in any question, any number of items, or all or none of them, may be correct. They are arranged under the chapter numbers of the current edition (6th Edition 1983) of *Lecture Notes on General Surgery*.

CHAPTER ONE

1. **Erysipelas**
   A  is a diffuse staphylococcal infection of the skin
   B  is a notifiable disease
   C  is characterized by necrosis of the subcutaneous tissue
   D  particularly occurs on the face and neck
   E  causes intense pain.

2. **Furuncles**

   A  commonly occur on the soles of the feet
   B  when multiple, should be treated by systemic chemotherapy
   C  are usually due to staphylococci
   D  are a recognized cause of cavernous sinus thrombosis if they occur on the face
   E  can cause osteomyelitis, usually by direct invasion of underlying bone.

3. **In tetanus**
    A   muscle spasm characteristically precedes the onset of the convulsions
    B   the patient nearly always loses consciousness during the convulsions
    C   the infection spreads along the muscle planes
    D   treatment with anti-tetanus serum is essential
    E   heavy sedation may be necessary to control the convulsions.

4. **Infection of an amputation stump with *Clostridium welchii***
    A   is associated with high fever throughout the course of the illness
    B   should be treated with penicillin
    C   produces a characteristic sensation on palpation of the affected part
    D   is an indication for hyperbaric oxygen therapy
    E   typically occurs several weeks after the amputation.

5. **The parts of the body characteristically affected by actinomycosis are**
    A   the ileo-caecal region
    B   the rectum and anal canal
    C   the jaw
    D   the spleen
    E   the lungs.

6. **Following acute haemorrhage**
    A   pallor and sweating are evidence of sympathetic overactivity
    B   the patient should be kept warm to restore skin blood flow

**C** the central venous pressure falls

**D** renal tubular necrosis is a recognized complication

**E** the degree of hypotension is a reliable index of the amount of blood lost.

## CHAPTER FOUR

**7. Superficial (partial thickness) burns**

    **A** are less painful than deep burns

    **B** usually heal without scarring

    **C** do not develop a slough

    **D** can be treated by either the 'open' or the 'closed' method

    **E** are associated with trivial exudation of plasma.

**8. In the treatment of burns**

    **A** shock is best treated by infusion of plasma

    **B** the mortality rate of burns of both legs and of the front of the trunk is about 50%

    **C** skin grafting is required if the slough has not separated after 2 weeks

    **D** exposure of a deep burn to the air is contraindicated

    **E** anaemia may be severe enough to require blood transfusion.

## CHAPTER FIVE

**9. In the postoperative period**

    **A** fatal pulmonary embolus is usually preceded by evidence of deep venous thrombosis in the legs

    **B** dehiscence of an abdominal wound is more likely to occur in patients who develop pulmonary collapse

    **C** thrombus usually begins to form in the leg veins in the second week

    **D** pseudo-membranous colitis should be treated with a broad-spectrum antibiotic

    **E** less than 1% of wounds become infected.

## CHAPTER SIX

10. **In the two or three days following anterior resection of the rectum in a man weighing 70 kg with previously normal renal function**
    A about 3 litres of fluid are required intravenously each 24 hours
    B corticosteroid secretion is typically depressed
    C sufficient dextrose should be given to provide about 1000 calories each 24 hours
    D hypokalaemia is often accompanied by metabolic alkalosis
    E excessive drainage from a nasogastric tube should be replaced by a similar amount of normal saline.

## CHAPTER EIGHT

11. **Fractures of the ribs**
    A most often occur in the upper three or four ribs
    B are unlikely to be complicated by pneumothorax unless the skin is broken
    C are best treated by firm strapping of the chest wall
    D cause pain which is aggravated by pressure on the sternum
    E most often occur in the posterior ends of the ribs.

12. **The immediate management of a severe chest injury should include**
    A firm support for the detached segment if a flail chest is present
    B bronchoscopy to exclude rupture of a bronchus
    C drainage of a tension pneumothorax, if present, via an underwater seal
    D surgical exploration if the venous pressure is rising and the blood pressure falling

**E** very light dressing of any penetrating wound to allow free escape of air from the pleural space.

13. **The association of haemoptysis and finger clubbing is suggestive of**
   **A** bronchial carcinoma
   **B** bronchiectasis
   **C** empyema
   **D** bronchial adenoma
   **E** pulmonary metastases.

14. **Recognized complications of bronchial carcinoma include**
   **A** peripheral neuropathy
   **B** atrial fibrillation
   **C** hoarseness of the voice
   **D** lung abscess
   **E** oedema and cyanosis of the face.

15. **Evidence of inoperability of a bronchial carcinoma includes**
   **A** palpable cervical lymph nodes
   **B** widening of the carina on bronchoscopy
   **C** malignant cells in the sputum
   **D** involvement of the chest wall
   **E** a respiratory infection persisting for longer than 2 weeks.

CHAPTER NINE

16. **Left ventricular hypertrophy is a recognized feature of**
   **A** persistent ductus arteriosus
   **B** Fallot's tetralogy
   **C** coarctation of the aorta
   **D** mitral stenosis
   **E** aortic stenosis.

17. **The following symptoms could reasonably be attributed to a syphilitic aneurysm of the aorta:**
    A  hoarseness
    B  sciatica
    C  haematuria
    D  dysphagia
    E  interscapular pain.

18. **Factors of importance in the aetiology of dissecting aneurysm include**
    A  hypertension
    B  fibromuscular hyperplasia of the aorta
    C  arteriosclerosis
    D  syphilis
    E  cystic medial necrosis of the aorta.

19. **Cardiopulmonary bypass, or profound hypothermia, is required for the surgical treatment of**
    A  coarctation of the aorta
    B  mitral stenosis
    C  aortic stenosis
    D  Fallot's tetralogy
    E  constrictive pericarditis.

CHAPTER TEN
20. **In a patient who has had an arterial embolism in a limb**
    A  it is important to keep the affected limb warm
    B  heparin should be given
    C  surgery is almost certainly required if the muscles of the limb are paralysed
    D  whenever possible surgery should be deferred for at least 24 hours

**E**  it is important to localize the embolus precisely so that the arteriotomy can be performed directly over it.

**21.  The features of Leriche's syndrome are**
   **A**  absent femoral pulses
   **B**  pain in the buttocks on walking
   **C**  pale cold legs
   **D**  a continuous bruit over the abdominal aorta
   **E**  impotence.

**22.  Intermittent claudication**
   **A**  should rarely be treated surgically if the patient has angina pectoris also
   **B**  can be expected to worsen inexorably in the great majority of patients
   **C**  can frequently be improved by lumbar sympathectomy
   **D**  is rarely worth treating by reconstructive surgery if arteriography shows that the popliteal artery is blocked
   **E**  may become less severe if the patient wears high-heeled shoes.

**23.  Raynaud's disease**
   **A**  affects females predominantly
   **B**  is characterized by cyanosis of the fingers immediately they are placed in cold water
   **C**  may affect the feet as well as the hands
   **D**  is usually strikingly improved by sympathectomy
   **E**  is usually associated with absent radial pulses.

24. **A woman aged 50 complains of the sudden onset of pain in the right arm. The limb is pale and cold and the radial pulse is absent. The following associated features are aetiologically significant:**

A  a recent myocardial infarction

B  mitral stenosis with atrial fibrillation

C  subacute bacterial endocarditis

D  atherosclerotic aneurysm of the descending thoracic aorta

E  cryoglobulinaemia.

CHAPTER ELEVEN

25. **Varicose (gravitational) ulcers**

A  may be preceded by a 'flare' of venules over the malleoli

B  should be treated with local antibiotics if infection has occurred

C  recur in about two-thirds of cases unless the associated varicose veins are treated effectively

D  are a recognized long-term result of deep venous thrombosis

E  are due to high pressure in the superficial veins.

26. **Varicose veins**

A  are due primarily to malfunction of the venous valves

B  are more common in females than in males

C  are due to a deep venous thrombosis when they occur in pregnancy

D  are most prominent where the superficial and deep venous systems communicate

E  can be emptied by vigorous contraction of the calf muscles.

## CHAPTER TWELVE

**27. Recognized causes of generalized lymphadenopathy include**

   **A** Hodgkin's disease

   **B** sarcoidosis

   **C** carcinomatosis

   **D** tuberculosis

   **E** secondary syphilis.

**28. Lymphoedema**

   **A** following surgery for malignant disease, implies that the tumour has recurred

   **B** may be present at birth

   **C** does not 'pit' on pressure and can thus be distinguished from oedema due to venous obstruction

   **D** is a recognized feature of filariasis

   **E** may be a sequel of X-ray therapy.

CHAPTER THIRTEEN

**29. A raised intracranial pressure**

   **A** is a recognized long-term sequel of meningitis

   **B** characteristically causes headache which is worse when the patient wakes

   **C** can be diagnosed by X-ray evidence of lateral displacement of the pineal

   **D** is an early manifestation of an acoustic tumour

   **E** is an important cause of papilloedema.

**30. The manifestations of an acoustic tumour include**

   **A** weakness of the facial muscles

   **B** nystagmus

   **C** motor aphasia

   **D** numbness of the face

   **E** tinnitus.

### 31. The following statements are correct:

A  Meningioma is the commonest intracranial tumour.

B  Medulloblastoma most often occurs in the cerebellum.

C  Calcification above the sella turcica seen in an X-ray is suggestive of craniopharyngioma.

D  Hyperostosis of the skull is a recognized feature of congenital hydrocephalus.

E  Most meningiomas can be removed completely.

### 32. Subarachnoid haemorrhage

A  is most often due to rupture of a congenital aneurysm

B  recurs in more than half the cases

C  has a good prognosis if no aneurysm can be demonstrated by angiography

D  has its peak incidence in the second decade of life

E  may be due to an angioma especially if there is a history of focal epilepsy.

CHAPTER FOURTEEN

### 33. In a patient who is unconscious following head injury

A  tachycardia and hypotension indicate increasing cerebral compression

B  changes in the level of consciousness are the most important guide to the need for surgery

C  if the pupils are unequal, a light shone into the dilated pupil will usually produce constriction of the opposite pupil

D  full recovery can be expected more often than not

E  a period of normal consciousness following the injury is suggestive of an extradural haemorrhage.

### 34. The physical signs of a fractured skull include

A  bleeding from the ear

**B** discharge of clear fluid from the nose, increased in amount by compression of the jugular veins

**C** a periorbital haematoma extending over the malar bone

**D** evidence of a lesion of one or more cranial nerves

**E** a subconjunctival haemorrhage at the outer canthus extending backwards out of sight.

## 35. Chronic subdural haematoma

**A** is preceded by a clear history of injury in nearly all cases

**B** enlarges as a result of recurrent bleeding over several weeks or months

**C** is bilateral in about 50% of cases

**D** can be delineated by CAT scanning

**E** commonly presents with headache and drowsiness.

## 36. Following head injury

**A** meningitis is a recognized complication

**B** hyperpyrexia may occur

**C** the longer the period of amnesia, the worse the prognosis

**D** epilepsy is a recognized long-term complication

**E** return to work may be delayed long after the time of full physical recovery.

CHAPTER FIFTEEN

## 37. Recognized features of myelomeningocele include

**A** loss of sphincter control

**B** a defect in the meninges

**C** talipes equinovarus

**D** hydrocephalus

**E** paraplegia.

38. **Following a fracture or dislocation of the spine**
   A permanent neurological damage is unlikely if the affected vertebra is 'wedged'
   B the stability of the fracture depends on the integrity of the supra-spinous ligament
   C full recovery is impossible if the cauda equina is injured
   D full recovery from a quadriplegia can be confidently expected if the lateral X-ray of the cervical spine is normal
   E the early evidence of cord transection includes flaccid paralysis, retention of urine and priapism.

39. **The features of prolapse of the disc between the fourth and fifth lumbar vertebrae include**
   A sciatic pain
   B sensory loss on the lateral side of the foot
   C weakness of dorsiflexion of the ankle
   D diminished ankle jerk
   E flattening of the normal lumbar lordosis.

40. **Recognized manifestations of spinal meningioma include**
   A pain in the distribution of one or more nerve roots
   B loss of position and vibration sense on the opposite side to the tumour
   C severe constipation
   D a combination of flaccid and spastic paralysis of muscles
   E rapid evolution of symptoms and signs.

CHAPTER SIXTEEN
41. **Following**
   A axonotmesis, full recovery of function of the nerve can be expected in a few days

**B** neurapraxia, regrowth of the axon occurs from the node of Ranvier proximal to the injury

**C** neurotmesis, full functional recovery is very unlikely

**D** complete severance of a nerve, the affected muscles no longer respond to any form of electrical stimulation

**E** division of a nerve in a contaminated wound, immediate suture is essential.

42. **Recognized features of a lesion of the lowermost root of the brachial plexus (Klumpke's paralysis) include**

  **A** assumption by the arm of the 'waiter's tip' position

  **B** wasting of the small muscles of the hand

  **C** loss of sensation over the medial side of the forearm

  **D** dilatation of the pupil

  **E** ptosis.

43. **On examination of the hand and wrist**

  **A** wrist drop is compatible with a lesion of the radial nerve

  **B** inability to abduct or adduct the fingers with the hand flat on a table is suggestive of a median nerve lesion

  **C** difficulty in doing needlework is more likely to be due to a lesion of the median nerve than of the ulnar nerve

  **D** weakness of flexion of the wrist could be due to the carpal tunnel syndrome

  **E** wasting of the thenar eminence is compatible with a median nerve lesion.

### 44. Flexion deformity of the fingers due to

**A** Volkmann's contracture can be relieved somewhat by flexion of the wrist

**B** Dupuytren's contracture involves the metacarpo-phalangeal and both interphalangeal joints

**C** congenital contracture causes trivial disability

**D** an ulnar nerve lesion is associated with sensory loss

**E** congenital contracture is usually bilateral.

CHAPTER SEVENTEEN

### 45. In the mouth, the following lesions are typically situated in the mid-line:

**A** ranula

**B** dermoid

**C** lingual thyroid

**D** mucous retention cyst

**E** carcinoma of the tongue.

### 46. Cleft lip

**A** is more often than not associated with a cleft palate

**B** occurs because of failure of fusion of the maxillary and mandibular processes

**C** should be repaired at 1 year to allow normal speech to develop

**D** predisposes to the development of carcinoma of the lip

**E** may rarely extend upwards along the side of the nose.

### 47. Carcinoma of the lip

**A** more often affects the lower lip than the upper

**B** metastasizes early to the internal jugular lymph nodes

C affects men more often than women

D has a poor prognosis if it occurs at the angle of the mouth

E is best treated by surgical excision.

## 48. Malignant disease of

A the tonsil most commonly arises in the lymphoid tissue

B the tongue can cause pain radiating to the ear

C the nasopharynx may present with deafness

D the floor of the mouth is most commonly an ulcerating squamous carcinoma

E the buccal mucosa can arise in a patch of leukoplakia.

CHAPTER EIGHTEEN

## 49. Carcinoma of the maxillary antrum

A is a recognized cause of epistaxis

B may present as acute sinusitis

C is typically resistant to radiotherapy

Ḋ affects both sexes equally

E can simulate cellulitis of the face.

CHAPTER NINETEEN

## 50. Salivary calculi

A are most common in the submandibular gland

B are always radio-opaque

C usually cause purulent discharge from the duct of the gland

D most commonly occur in patients with gross dental caries

E should be suspected if the patient complains of an unpleasant taste.

51. **A pleomorphic adenoma ('mixed tumour') of the parotid gland**
    A   occurs most often in patients over the age of 50
    B   tends to recur after local enucleation
    C   characteristically contains cartilage
    D   causes facial paralysis in about 50% of cases
    E   lies within a fibrous capsule.

52. **A patient presents with a swelling of one parotid gland. The following features will be helpful in determining the nature of the swelling:**
    A   facial paralysis
    B   a history of recent major surgery
    C   dehydration
    D   pain in the gland after meals
    E   a mass projecting into the pharynx.

CHAPTER TWENTY
53. **Dysphagia may result from**
    A   multiple sclerosis
    B   myasthenia gravis
    C   bulbar palsy
    D   tabes dorsalis
    E   poliomyelitis.

54. **The most likely cause of dysphagia**
    A   in an elderly male is carcinoma of the oesophagus
    B   is simple stricture if there is a history of reflux oesophagitis
    C   in a young female with progressive severe weight loss is achalasia
    D   is a foreign body if there is pain on swallowing
    E   in an infant of 2 weeks is oesophageal atresia.

## 55. Carcinoma of the oesophagus
A may present with hepatomegaly and jaundice
B nearly always arises in squamous epithelium
C usually gives no striking abnormality on barium swallow
D is best treated by resection especially if the upper level of the tumour reaches above the aortic arch
E responds uniformly badly to radiotherapy.

## CHAPTER TWENTY-ONE

## 56. Reflux oesophagitis
A can cause pain radiating to the jaw and arms
B is more likely to occur with a 'rolling' than with a 'sliding' hiatal hernia
C is a recognized cause of chronic anaemia
D causes pain which is usually relieved by rest in bed
E does not occur in the absence of a hiatal hernia.

## 57. Congenital diaphragmatic herniae can occur through
A a foramen closely related to the xiphoid
B a congenitally large oesophageal hiatus
C a persistent pleuroperitoneal canal
D the hiatus in the diaphragm for the inferior vena cava
E a defect in the septum transversum.

## CHAPTER TWENTY-TWO

## 58. Congenital hypertrophic pyloric stenosis
A is a condition of unknown aetiology
B only rarely occurs in siblings
C typically presents within a day or two of birth
D demands a few days preoperative preparation in severe cases
E responds as well to atropine methylnitrate as to operation.

### 59. In an infant suffering from persistent vomiting
   **A** the presence of bile in the vomit is compatible with duodenal atresia
   **B** the absence of bile in the vomit favours the diagnosis of pyloric stenosis
   **C** a plain X-ray of the abdomen is unlikely to provide diagnostic help
   **D** duodenal atresia is more likely if the child is a mongol
   **E** rehydration and gastric aspiration should be undertaken before an attempt at surgical relief.

### 60. Acute peptic ulceration of the stomach may be related to
   **A** acute stress
   **B** ingestion of alcohol
   **C** treatment with indomethacin
   **D** severe burns
   **E** a major operation.

### 61. Chronic duodenal ulcer
   **A** will usually respond to treatment with cimetidine
   **B** is associated with vitamin D deficiency
   **C** is extremely unlikely to be present in a patient who is gaining weight
   **D** is best treated surgically by a Billroth I gastrectomy
   **E** is rare in premenopausal women.

### 62. Perforation of an anterior duodenal ulcer
   **A** is most likely to be encountered in teenage females
   **B** is more likely to occur in patients on chronic corticosteroid treatment
   **C** causes pain which is aggravated by movement
   **D** is commonly confused with coronary thrombosis
   **E** carries a mortality of less than 1%.

63. **Recognized metabolic changes in patients with chronic duodenal ulceration leading to 'pyloric stenosis' include**
   A  alkalosis due to loss of hydrogen ions in the vomit
   B  compensatory increased renal excretion of sodium bicarbonate
   C  an acid urine, even in the presence of advanced alkalosis
   D  a fall in the concentration of calcium ions in the plasma
   E  increased renal excretion of chloride.


64. **In patients presenting with acute gastrointestinal haemorrhage**
   A  four out of five are likely to be suffering from peptic ulceration
   B  physical examination usually provides diagnostic information on the likely cause of bleeding
   C  immediate haemoglobin estimation provides useful information on the extent of bleeding
   D  mortality is higher in patients over 45
   E  gastrotomy should be performed if the source of the bleeding is not immediately obvious at laparotomy.


65. **Carcinoma of the stomach**
   A  is the third commonest carcinoma in males in Britain
   B  is commoner in patients with a high alcoholic consumption
   C  is commoner in patients of blood group O
   D  can usually be shown to have arisen in a previously benign lesion
   E  is always an adenocarcinoma, with varying degrees of differentiation.

## CHAPTER TWENTY-THREE

**66. In a case of mechanical intestinal obstruction**

    **A** strangulation implies that the blood supply to the involved segment of intestine is cut off

    **B** strangulated hernia should be seriously considered at any age

    **C** absolute constipation is invariable

    **D** the bowel beyond the obstruction becomes collapsed

    **E** perforation of the intestine will not occur in the absence of external pressure on the bowel.

**67. The following principles apply in the treatment of mechanical intestinal obstruction:**

    **A** Chronic large bowel obstruction can be investigated at leisure and treated electively even if plain X-ray of the abdomen shows a dilated caecum.

    **B** However urgent the need for surgery in acute obstruction, naso-gastric suction and intravenous replacement of fluid and electrolytes should be undertaken preoperatively.

    **C** Antibiotics are indicated if there is a possibility of intestinal strangulation.

    **D** A purple segment of bowel is not viable.

    **E** A segment of small bowel can be resected with greater safety than a segment of large bowel.

## CHAPTER TWENTY-FOUR

**68. In a case of neonatal intestinal obstruction**

    **A** a gush of flatus and faeces after rectal examination suggests Hirschsprung's disease

    **B** anorectal atresia is only rarely associated with fistula into vagina, urethra or bladder

C a plain X-ray of the abdomen will have a typical appearance in meconium ileus

D volvulus is usually due to adhesions

E projectile vomiting of bile-free material is characteristic.

**69. Volvulus**

A is defined as a twisting of a loop of bowel around its mesenteric axis

B of the sigmoid usually occurs in elderly constipated men

C does not occur in the stomach

D of the small intestine is commoner in Africa than in Britain

E is more likely to occur in the presence of an abnormally mobile loop of intestine.

CHAPTER TWENTY-FIVE

**70. Meckel's diverticulum**

A may be responsible for ileal volvulus

B can cause an umbilical fistula

C should be considered in patients presenting with the clinical picture of acute appendicitis

D occurs about 5 feet proximal to the ileo-caecal valve

E does not lead to intestinal bleeding.

**71. Crohn's disease**

A may affect the oesophagus

B only affects the colon if the ileum is involved too

C has been thought to be due to an autoimmune reaction

D affects the whole thickness of the bowel wall

E causes a characteristic cobblestone appearance of the mucous membrane.

72. **The carcinoid syndrome should be considered in patients in whom there is**
   A   obstinate constipation
   B   unexplained attacks of profuse sweating
   C   an unexpected aortic valve lesion
   D   a combination of hepatic enlargement and broncho-spasm
   E   a pink discolouration of the urine after it has been allowed to stand for a few hours.

CHAPTER TWENTY-SIX

73. **Acute appendicitis**
   A   is only prevalent in people taking a Western diet
   B   may occur in a non-obstructed appendix
   C   produces pain which is referred to the right iliac fossa irrespective of the anatomical position of the tip of the appendix.
   D   gives pain which causes the patient to writhe about
   E   has a higher mortality in pregnancy.

74. **The differential diagnosis of acute appendicitis includes**
   A   pneumonia
   B   herpes zoster
   C   ectopic pregnancy
   D   pericarditis
   E   renal colic.

75. **Conservative treatment of acute appendicitis should be undertaken**
   A   if the patient has had pain for more than 48 hours

**B** if the patient is moribund
**C** if general peritonitis is present
**D** if there is a localized mass in the right iliac fossa
**E** if there is a remission of pain, however short.

## CHAPTER TWENTY-SEVEN

**76. It is not surprising to find diarrhoea in a patient**
   **A** on morphine
   **B** on digitalis
   **C** who has had a vagotomy
   **D** who is uraemic
   **E** who has myxoedema.

**77. Colonic diverticula**
   **A** are commoner in the right than in the left side of the colon
   **B** are not usually found under the age of 40
   **C** occur much more commonly in females
   **D** are rare among primitive peoples
   **E** are preceded by atrophy of colonic muscle.

**78. Diverticular disease of the colon**
   **A** may result in the passage of bright red blood per rectum
   **B** is the commonest cause of vesico-colic fistula
   **C** is easy to distinguish from carcinoma on barium enema
   **D** may lead to small intestinal obstruction even in patients who have not been treated surgically
   **E** usually demands a defunctioning colostomy if surgical treatment is undertaken.

27

### 79. Carcinoma of the colon

**A** occurs more commonly in the transverse colon than in the sigmoid

**B** may spread via the thoracic duct to supraclavicular lymph nodes

**C** invariably develops in patients suffering from familial polyposis coli unless they are treated surgically

**D** occurs in more than 50% of cases of ulcerative colitis of 20 years' duration

**E** is more likely to cause intestinal obstruction if the tumour is in the ascending colon.

## CHAPTER TWENTY-EIGHT

### 80. Internal haemorrhoids

**A** usually occur at 6, 8 and 10 o'clock with a patient in the lithotomy position

**B** when persistently prolapsed outside the anal margin are classified as second degree haemorrhoids

**C** may be precipitated by pregnancy

**D** cause pain even in the absence of thrombosis

**E** are easily felt per rectum.

### 81. Haemorrhoidectomy

**A** is obligatory for thrombosed strangulated piles

**B** may lead to acute retention of urine

**C** causes secondary haemorrhage which may not be easily recognized

**D** is the treatment of choice for second degree piles

**E** should not be undertaken before excluding a predisposing cause of piles.

### 82. The following statements about anal disease are correct:

**A** Early surgical drainage of an ano-rectal abscess reduces the incidence of fistula-in-ano.

**B** Stretching of the anal sphincter helps an anal fissure to heal by paralysing the muscle temporarily.

**C** A perianal haematoma (thrombosed external pile) does not subside spontaneously in less than 2 weeks.

**D** Surgical treatment of a submucous fistula-in-ano carries a risk of faecal incontinence.

**E** Anal stricture may be due to lymphogranuloma inguinale.

## 83. Carcinoma of the rectum

**A** is an adenocarcinoma in 90% of cases

**B** has a prognosis which varies with the histological degree of differentiation

**C** may give rise to enlarged inguinal lymph nodes

**D** may give physical signs per rectum which can be confused with those produced by an IUD (intra-uterine contraceptive device)

**E** needs to be differentiated from amoebic granuloma.

CHAPTER TWENTY-NINE

## 84. Tuberculous peritonitis

**A** is becoming commoner in Britain

**B** can be excluded if there are signs of free fluid in the abdomen

**C** may present with intestinal obstruction

**D** can usually be controlled by antituberculous chemotherapy

**E** may complicate generalized miliary tuberculosis.

## 85. A swinging temperature after apparent recovery from peritonitis requires

**A** a white cell count

**B** rectal examination

**C** intravenous cholangiogram

**D** X-ray screening of the chest

**E** lung scan.

### 86. Paralytic ileus

A  gives rise to abdominal distension

B  may complicate a fracture of the pelvis

C  may be caused by heavy dosage with anticholinergic agents

D  occurs as a result of hyperkalaemia in acute renal failure

E  is to be expected for 1 or 2 days after any abdominal operation.

### 87. The following are features of paralytic ileus which help to distinguish it from mechanical intestinal obstruction:

A  persistence of symptoms for more than 4 days

B  severe pain

C  the absence of bowel sounds

D  severe electrolyte depletion

E  diffuse gas shadows throughout the bowel on a plain abdominal X-ray.

CHAPTER THIRTY-ONE

### 88. Factors which predisopose to the formation of a hernia include

A  persistence of the processus vaginalis

B  postoperative haematoma in the abdominal wall

C  chronic cough

D  regular vigorous exercise

E  gross obesity.

### 89. The inguinal canal

A  transmits the ilio-inguinal nerve

B  is covered anteriorly in its full length by the external oblique aponeurosis

C is covered anteriorly in its medial third by the conjoint tendon

D ends at the external ring immediately above and medial to the pubic tubercle

E lies anterior to the external iliac vessels.

90. **An inguinal hernia is more likely to be indirect than direct if it**
   A appears immediately on standing
   B is strangulated
   C presents in adolescence
   D can be completely controlled by pressure with a finger tip over the internal inguinal ring
   E has a cough impulse.

91. **The following statements about hernias are correct:**
   A Ventral hernia usually requires no treatment.
   B Congenital umbilical hernia should be repaired surgically before the child is 2 years old.
   C Epigastric hernia, though it only contains extraperitoneal fat, is often painful.
   D Incisional hernia is extremely likely to strangulate.
   E Obturator hernia may produce pain along the medial side of the thigh.

CHAPTER THIRTY-TWO
92. **A palpable liver**
   A may be normal
   B may be due to polycystic disease
   C if accompanied by a palpable spleen, suggests cirrhosis as a possible diagnosis
   D if lymph nodes and spleen are also felt, suggests hydatid disease
   E is improbable in infective hepatitis.

### 93. In a case of jaundice

A  a family history of anaemia may give a clue to the diagnosis

B  enquiry about drugs is important

C  a history of severe pain and rigors suggests viral hepatitis

D  continuous pain radiating to the back suggests malignant disease

E  tenderness of the liver is strongly suggestive of cirrhosis.

### 94. In the metabolism of bile pigments

A  the porphyrin ring of the haemoglobin molecule is the source of bilirubin-iron-globin complex

B  bilirubin is rendered water-soluble by conjugation with glucuronic acid

C  the normal stool colour is due to the presence of urobilinogen

D  some urobilinogen is normally reabsorbed from the gut and excreted by the kidneys

E  bilirubin is excreted in the urine in a lipid-soluble form.

### 95. In the investigation of a case of jaundice

A  a prolonged prothrombin time can be corrected in the presence of post-hepatic obstruction

B  the level of alkaline phosphatase gives no diagnostic help

C  needle biopsy of the liver is dangerous

D  plain abdominal X-ray will show gall stones, if present, in 90% of cases

E  a cholecystogram is more helpful than a barium meal.

### 96. Hydatid disease of the liver

A  should be treated surgically if the cyst is calcified

**B** is acquired from vegetables contaminated by the faeces of dogs

**C** is common in Iceland

**D** may produce obstructive jaundice

**E** may be diagnosed by a complement fixation test even after the death of the parasite.

**97. In hepatic cirrhosis**

**A** alcohol is the commonest aetiological factor in the USA

**B** the severity of the liver disease has a strict relationship to the extent of portal hypertension

**C** the development of collateral channels between the left gastric and oesophageal veins has more clinical significance than retroperitoneal anastomoses

**D** splenomegaly is often associated with leucocytosis

**E** ascites is partly due to increased aldosterone activity.

**98. Important elements in the management of haemorrhage from oesophageal varices include**

**A** blood transfusion

**B** high protein diet

**C** intramuscular neomycin

**D** intravenous pitressin

**E** the passage of a Sengstaken tube.

CHAPTER THIRTY-THREE

**99. Gall stones**

**A** are present in about 10% of patients over 40

**B** occur in children suffering from haemolytic anaemia

**C** produce severe pain rising to a plateau and lasting for many hours

**D** may be present in the common bile duct even if there are no symptoms

**E** should be removed surgically if the patient is young and symptomless.

**100. In acute cholecystitis**

    **A** jaundice does not occur unless gall stones are present

    **B** cholecystectomy is best performed about 1 week after the onset of the illness

    **C** leucocytosis is a recognized feature

    **D** suppurative cholangitis is a common complication

    **E** a tender mass can often be felt in the upper abdomen.

CHAPTER THIRTY-FOUR

**101. Heterotopic pancreatic tissue**

    **A** occurs in over 50% of people

    **B** arises from the primitive midgut

    **C** may be found in the jejunum

    **D** is particularly liable to be affected by pancreatitis

    **E** may cause intestinal obstruction.

**102. Acute pancreatitis**

    **A** is typically associated with bile-stained ascites

    **B** gives rise to fat necrosis only in previously hypercalcaemic patients

    **C** causes severe constant epigastric pain

    **D** is very unlikely to cause fever

    **E** produces glycosuria in about 4 cases out of 5.

**103. In the treatment of acute pancreatitis**

    **A** pain should be relieved by morphine

    **B** blood transfusion may be required

    **C** antibiotics have no place

    **D** calcium gluconate may be required

    **E** surgery should not be undertaken unless the diagnosis is certain.

**104. Chronic relapsing pancreatitis may present with**

A diabetes mellitus

B obstructive jaundice

C gross ascites

D recurrent pain in the back

E gastrointestinal haemorrhage.

**105. True pancreatic cysts**

A are commoner than pseudocysts

B follow acute pancreatitis

C are dull to percussion even if quite small

D may be due to hydatid disease

E require surgical excision.

**106. In a case of carcinoma of the pancreas**

A it is unusual for pain to occur before jaundice is evident

B once jaundice occurs, it inevitably progresses without remission

C the liver may be enlarged even in the absence of hepatic metastases

D thrombophlebitis migrans may be the presenting feature

E barium meal examination is often completely negative, even in the presence of advanced disease.

CHAPTER THIRTY-FIVE

**107. Massive splenomegaly in the UK is likely to be due to**

A glandular fever

B polycythaemia

C chronic leukaemia

D malaria

E portal hypertension.

**108. Splenectomy is indicated**
   A in the course of spleno-renal anastomosis
   B for hydatid disease of the spleen
   C in amyloid disease
   D for thrombocytopenic purpura
   E for splenic rupture.

**109. If rupture of the spleen is suspected**
   A it is important to percuss carefully in the left flank
   B the absence of bruising of the abdominal wall virtually excludes the condition
   C observation can be safely discontinued if there has been no deterioration for 4 hours
   D the urine should always be tested for blood
   E X-rays of the abdomen are of little or no value.

CHAPTER THIRTY-SIX

**110. The following statements about congenital renal anomalies are correct:**
   A Variations in the renal blood supply are rare.
   B Pelvic kidney is due to failure of its cranial migration during development.
   C Double ureters are due to reduplication of the metanephric bud.
   D Polycystic kidneys are probably due to failure of linkage between the mesonephric duct and the mesonephros.
   E Congenital hydronephrosis does not depend on anatomical malformation.

**111. Polycystic disease of the kidneys**
   A may be associated with cysts in the liver and pancreas
   B is carried by a dominant gene
   C more often presents with renal failure than with haematuria

**D** is a possible cause of hypertensive heart failure

**E** only rarely permits survival beyond the age of 40.

### 112. In a patient with haematuria

**A** it is particularly important to take a drug history

**B** the presence of pain makes a tumour very unlikely

**C** examination of the heart may give a clue to the cause

**D** it is important to examine the urine microscopically

**E** cystoscopy should not be undertaken until bleeding has stopped.

### 113. In a case of injury to the kidney

**A** there is usually a history of a penetrating wound

**B** abdominal distension due to ileus may occur

**C** conservative management is usually all that is required

**D** severe persistent hypertension is a contraindication to nephrectomy

**E** intravenous pyelography is of little value.

### 114. Hydronephrosis

**A** does not cause pain unless calculi are present

**B** predisposes to the formation of calculi

**C** may present with rigors

**D** is a recognized cause of hypertension

**E** may be due to tuberculosis.

### 115. The following factors predispose to the formation of calculi in the urinary tract:

**A** paraplegia

**B** prostatic hypertrophy

**C** anaemia

**D** hyperparathyroidism

**E** residence in the tropics.

### 116. A ureteric calculus

A produces pain which is best treated initially with pethidine

B may lodge at the point where the ureter crosses the pelvic brim

C should be treated by reduction of fluid intake

D can only be removed by the Dormia basket if the stone is seen at cystoscopy to be lodged at the ureteric orifice

E usually passes spontaneously.

### 117. Indications for surgery in renal tuberculosis include

A extensive fibrosis of the bladder

B unilateral irregularity of calyces on intravenous pyelogram

C pyonephrosis

D failure to sterilize the urine after 2 months chemotherapeutic treatment

E concomitant pulmonary tuberculosis.

### 118. In a case of nephroblastoma (Wilm's tumour)

A the patient is usually less than 4 years old

B muscle fibres may be found on histological examination of the tumour

C haematuria is to be expected

D preoperative radiotherapy may be of some value if the tumour is very large

E cytotoxic therapy has nothing to offer.

### 119. Adenocarcinoma of the kidney (hypernephroma)

A originates from renal tubules

B tends to spread down the ureter

C can cause pain even in the absence of clot colic

D should not be treated surgically if a pulmonary metastasis is found

E may present as a pyrexia of unknown origin (PUO).

## CHAPTER THIRTY-SEVEN

**120. Rupture of the bladder**

   **A** does not occur unless the bladder has been traumatized

   **B** is probably extraperitoneal if there is a swelling arising out of the pelvis

   **C** is easier to suture if the rupture is extraperitoneal

   **D** should always be treated by drainage of the retropubic space even if the rupture cannot be repaired

   **E** may occur as a result of repair of a hernia.

**121. A bladder stone**

   **A** is likely to arise in a paraplegic patient

   **B** causes frequency of micturition which is worse by day

   **C** characteristically causes pain as soon as the patient starts to empty his bladder

   **D** is difficult to demonstrate on a straight X-ray

   **E** may consist of calcium oxalate.

**122. Factors which favour the development of a tumour of the bladder include**

   **A** increasing age

   **B** the presence of a diverticulum

   **C** heavy smoking

   **D** chronic malaria

   **E** schistosomiasis.

**123. Carcinoma of the bladder**

   **A** is usually very painful in the early stages

   **B** is usually accompanied by haematuria

   **C** most often occurs in the vault of the bladder

   **D** is best diagnosed by cystoscopy

   **E** has a good prognosis, once surgery has been undertaken.

## CHAPTER THIRTY-EIGHT

**124. Benign enlargement of the prostate**

A  only becomes common after the age of 65

B  may cause elongation of the prostatic urethra

C  acts like a ball valve when the median lobe is affected

D  may cause frequency of micturition even in the absence of urinary tract infection

E  is a similar condition to chronic mastitis in the female.

**125. Retention of urine due to benign prostatic enlargement**

A  is sometimes painless

B  makes the gland feel smaller than it really is on rectal examination

C  is a contraindication to intravenous pyelography

D  is nearly always associated with urinary tract infection

E  is best treated initially by carbachol.

**126. Carcinoma of the prostate**

A  is rare below the age of 50

B  is sometimes anaplastic

C  is suggested by the abolition of the sulcus between the two lobes on rectal examination

D  metastasizes to the inguinal lymph nodes

E  is typically associated with osteolytic bony metastases.

**127. In the treatment of prostatic carcinoma**

A  patients are, on the whole, consistent in their response to oestrogens

B  100 mg of stilboestrol daily is the usual starting dose

C fluid retention may limit effective oestrogen dosage
D bilateral orchidectomy is indicated if oestrogen treatment cannot be undertaken
E radiotherapy may relieve the pain of bony deposits.

## CHAPTER THIRTY-NINE

## 128. Congenital abnormalities of the urethra
A are confined to the male
B interfere with potency
C interfere with fertility
D may lead to uraemia in infants
E predispose to rupture of the urethra.

## 129. A patient with a urethral stricture
A usually gives a previous history of syphilis
B may have had a previous causally-related blow on the perineum
C finds that straining helps him to empty the bladder
D is best treated by monthly dilatation with sounds
E should be given long-term treatment with anti-biotics if the lesion is infective in origin.

## CHAPTER FORTY

## 130. Ammoniacal dermatitis
A should be treated by reducing the frequency of changing of nappies so as to avoid further chafing of the skin
B should be treated by circumcision in order to avoid the development of a meatal ulcer
C is more likely to occur in uraemic infants
D should be treated by local disinfectant solutions
E predisposes to carcinoma of the penis later in life.

## CHAPTER FORTY-ONE

**131. An undescended testis**

    **A**  is usually associated with pituitary hypofunction

    **B**  should be fixed in the scrotum operatively before the age of 7

    **C**  is commonly easily palpable in the groin

    **D**  is more likely than a normally situated testis to undergo torsion

    **E**  is associated with persistence of the processus vaginalis.

**132. Malignant disease of the testis**

    **A**  is a recognized complication of maldescent of the testis

    **B**  is most common over the age of 50

    **C**  is associated with gynaecomastia in the majority of cases

    **D**  should be treated routinely by radiotherapy to the abdomen as well as orchidectomy

    **E**  may be diagnosed as a result of routine chest radiography.

## CHAPTER FORTY-TWO

**133. Tuberculous cervical adenitis**

    **A**  is usually secondary to a primary focus in a tonsil

    **B**  characteristically causes a bilocular abscess

    **C**  is often associated with typical X-ray appearances

    **D**  requires surgical removal of the primary focus as well as anti-tuberculous chemotherapy

    **E**  is almost always due to drinking infected milk.

## CHAPTER FORTY-THREE

**134. Thyroid stimulating hormone (TSH)**

    **A**  production is greater than normal in patients with colloid goitre

**B** production can be suppressed by the administration of carbimazole

**C** secretion is under the influence of thyrotrophin-releasing hormone secreted by the hypothalamus

**D** is secreted by the posterior lobe of the pituitary

**E** stimulates the release of tri-iodothyronine and thyroxine from the thyroid.

135. **Radio-iodine studies are of value in the investigation of suspected**

A colloid goitre

B lingual thyroid

C thyroid carcinoma

D toxic nodular goitre

E thyroglossal fistula.

136. **Factors which determine the choice of treatment for thyrotoxicosis include**

A the age of the patient

B the high relapse rate after carbimazole therapy

C the potentially serious side-effects of carbimazole

D the high incidence of late myxoedema after radio-iodine therapy

E the high incidence of thyroid crisis after thyroidectomy in severe cases.

137. **Recognized long and short term complications of thyroidectomy include**

A mania and hyperpyrexia

B aphonia

C stridor

D cataracts

E carpopedal spasm.

## 138. Carcinoma of the thyroid

A has a very poor prognosis in elderly patients

B is easily confused clinically with Hashimoto's disease

C should be treated with thyroxine, whatever other treatment is given

D sometimes consists of cells which secrete calcitonin

E if well-differentiated, has a good prognosis unless the regional lymph nodes are involved.

CHAPTER FORTY-FOUR

## 139. The metabolic effects of hyperparathyroidism include

A hypercalciuria

B hypophosphaturia

C raised serum alkaline phosphatase

D metabolic alkalosis

E hyperphosphataemia

CHAPTER FORTY-FIVE

## 140. Recognized features of phaeochromocytoma include

A pallor

B hypoglycaemia

C sustained hypertension

D palpitation

E blurring of vision.

CHAPTER FORTY-SIX

## 141. Recognized features of Cushing's syndrome include

A pallor

B hypertension

C menorrhagia

D diabetes mellitus

E osteoporosis.

## 142. The congenital form of the adrenogenital syndrome

A is usually due to a defect of corticosteroid synthesis

**B** should be treated by bilateral adrenalectomy

**C** is a cause of female pseudohermaphroditism

**D** causes delay in epiphyseal fusion

**E** is a recognized cause of acute adrenocortical insufficiency.

## CHAPTER FORTY-EIGHT

**143. In a patient with a solid lump in the breast**

    **A** tethering of the lump to the skin is pathognomonic of carcinoma

    **B** a diagnosis of fat necrosis should not be made unless there is a history of trauma

    **C** excision biopsy is mandatory

    **D** associated blood-stained discharge from the nipple is strongly suggestive of carcinoma

    **E** premenstrual pain in the lump is suggestive of localized chronic mastitis.

**144. The TNM classification of a breast cancer is influenced by**

    **A** the fixity of enlarged axillary lymph nodes

    **B** the size of the tumour

    **C** the size of the axillary lymph nodes

    **D** ulceration of the skin

    **E** the histological appearance of the tumour.

**145. In chronic mastitis**

    **A** the large cysts are the most characteristic feature after the menopause

    **B** carcinoma may develop in the wall of a cyst

    **C** infiltration with polymorphs is a characteristic histological finding

    **D** palpation with the flat of the hand reveals a characteristic 'lumpiness'

    **E** axillary lymph nodes may be palpable.

**146. Surgical cure of carcinoma of the breast cannot be expected if**
   A   there is indrawing of the nipple
   B   the tumour is fixed to the pectoral muscles
   C   there is associated Paget's disease of the nipple
   D   the axillary lymph nodes are fixed
   E   the disease occurs during pregnancy

CHAPTER FORTY-NINE
**147. The sole of the foot is a common site of**
   A   verruca vulgaris
   B   intradermal naevus (common mole)
   C   malignant melanoma
   D   sebaceous cyst
   E   lipoma.

**148. A valuable clue to the nature of a lesion on the hand or fingers may be provided by**
   A   exquisite tenderness
   B   the fact that the patient is elderly
   C   a healed scar over the lesion
   D   the fact that the patient is a hairdresser
   E   growth of the lesion to an inch in diameter in a few weeks.

**149. Malignant melanomata**
   A   are found only in the skin
   B   give rise to cutaneous nodules proximally in the affected limb
   C   most commonly arise from pre-existent intradermal naevi
   D   are the most common malignant tumours of the skin
   E   should be treated by wide local excision.

**150. The following statements are correct:**

A   Severe pain in a varicose ulcer suggests that malignant change has occurred.

B   Early spread to the regional lymph nodes is a characteristic feature of basal cell carcinoma.

C   Senile keratosis is a recognized precursor of squamous cell carcinoma.

D   Strawberry naevi usually disappear spontaneously.

E   Kaposi's sarcoma is a malignant tumour of vascular endothelium.

CHAPTER FIFTY

**151. The following factors determine the success of renal transplantation:**

A   The relationship between donor and recipient.

B   The use of high-potency anti-lymphocyte globulin in large doses.

C   Carefully regulated dosage of azathioprine.

D   Removal of the kidney from a cadaver donor within one hour of death.

E   The closeness of the matching between recipient and a related donor for HL-A antigens.

# PART TWO

The questions in this section are of the *Independent True/False* type, i.e. the same type as those in Part 1.

1. **Hyperparathyroidism**
   A  may result from renal disease
   B  is a recognized cause of symptoms very similar to those of gastric carcinoma
   C  causes a rise in serum calcium which falls to normal if cortisone is given for 10 days
   D  is a recognized cause of tetany
   E  causes bony decalcification associated with increased osteoclastic activity.

2. **A malignant tumour is the usual cause of**
   A  Cushing's syndrome
   B  carcinoid syndrome
   C  paroxysmal hypertension
   D  hyperparathyroidism
   E  myasthenia gravis.

3. **A strong clue to the nature of a mediastinal mass seen in the chest X-ray would be provided by**
   A  café-au-lait patches on the skin
   B  intermittent ptosis and diplopia
   C  long-standing dysphagia
   D  aortic regurgitation
   E  hoarseness of the voice.

**4. Carcinoma of the following organs characteristically metastasizes to the bones:**
A prostate
B rectum
C thyroid
D breast
E lung.

**5. A faecal fistula following hemi-colectomy**
A is associated with very rapid excoriation of the skin
B requires treatment with prolonged intravenous feeding
C is more likely to occur if the remaining distal bowel is obstructed
D is an unpredictable complication, unrelated to the general condition of the patient
E can sometimes usefully be fitted with a colostomy appliance.

**6. Stilboestrol has a place in the treatment of**
A the adrenogenital syndrome
B carcinoma of the breast
C carcinoma of the prostate
D seminoma of the testis
E teratoma of the testis.

**7. Recognized causes of urinary retention include**
A spinal meningioma
B urethral stricture
C carcinoma of the penis
D diverticulum of the bladder
E uterine fibroids.

8. **Metastases in the lymph nodes of the groin are a recognized feature of**
   - **A** carcinoma of the anal margin
   - **B** carcinoma of the bladder
   - **C** carcinoma of the penis
   - **D** melanoma of the buttock
   - **E** seminoma of the testis.

9. **Tissue necrosis is a characteristic feature of**
   - **A** Raynaud's disease
   - **B** carbuncle
   - **C** tetanus
   - **D** strangulated hernia
   - **E** severe amoebic hepatitis.

10. **The following occur at least twice as often in males as in females:**
    - **A** hiatal hernia
    - **B** ulcerative colitis
    - **C** diverticulum of bladder
    - **D** duodenal ulcer
    - **E** congenital hypertrophic pyloric stenosis.

11. **Recognized complications of urethral catheterization include**
    - **A** phimosis
    - **B** acute pyelonephritis
    - **C** urethral stricture
    - **D** paraphimosis
    - **E** carbuncle of the kidney.

12. **Recognized causes of lung abscess include**
    - **A** inhalation of a peanut

   **B** cerebral abscess
   **C** staphylococcal septicaemia
   **D** bronchial carcinoma
   **E** pulmonary infarction.

**13. Chromophobe adenoma of the pituitary**
   **A** is a recognized cause of bitemporal hemianopia
   **B** is the most common pituitary tumour
   **C** is a recognized cause of Cushing's syndrome
   **D** occurs in the remnant of the craniopharyngeal duct
   **E** is a recognized cause of hypothyroidism.

**14. A man aged 65 is admitted to hospital unconscious following a car accident in which he suffered a head injury.**
   **A** The finding of hemiparesis is a clear indication for surgical exploration.
   **B** Restlessness should be controlled with morphine.
   **C** It is important to exclude cerebral oedema by observing the effect of intravenous mannitol before proceeding to surgery.
   **D** Nasogastric feeding should be started if the patient is unable to swallow after 12 hours.
   **E** It is essential to X-ray the skull.

**15. Actinomycosis**
   **A** characteristically involves the regional lymph nodes
   **B** may follow the chewing of contaminated straw
   **C** is a recognized cause of sinus formation
   **D** causes the production of pus containing yellow specks
   **E** produces a soft fluctuant mass in the affected region.

16. **An aneurysm of the abdominal aorta**
    A  is often visible on plain X-ray of the abdomen
    B  is very unlikely to rupture unless it has caused pain in the back
    C  is usually saccular
    D  should be treated surgically if there is good evidence that it is enlarging.
    E  should usually be delineated by aortography before advising surgical treatment.

17. **Likely causes of a swelling in the region of the lower jaw near its angle include**
    A  ameloblastoma (adamantinoma)
    B  osteoclastoma
    C  congenital cyst
    D  leontiasis ossea
    E  actinomycosis.

18. **A diagnosis of carcinoma of the stomach**
    A  should be suspected if barium meal shows an ulcer over 2 cm in diameter
    B  should still be considered even after serial X-rays have shown considerable healing of a gastric ulcer
    C  is much easier to make if gastric acid secretion has been measured after pentagastrin administration
    D  may be made by finding malignant cells in a smear taken through a gastroscope
    E  may be suggested by symptoms identical with those of uraemia.

19. **Mesenteric vascular occlusion should be strongly suspected as the cause of colicky abdominal pain in a patient with**
    A  atrial fibrillation
    B  atheroma

C a history of recent splenectomy

D recent myocardial infarction

E hepatic cirrhosis.

## 20. In a case of Crohn's disease

A postoperative malabsorption may be due to the production of blind loops of intestine, quite apart from the extent of resection

B recurrence of the disease after resection may be expected in about 50% of cases within 10 years

C treatment should be surgical only in the case of severe obstruction

D steroids have a part to play in the control of acute episodes

E surgery does not increase the risk of development of an external faecal fistula.

## 21. In a case of peritonitis

A absolute constipation is to be expected

B pneumococcal septicaemia may be the underlying cause

C collapse of the lung may result from elevation of the diaphragm

D diagnosis is greatly helped by a plain X-ray of the abdomen

E there is usually a marked leucocytosis.

## 22. A femoral hernia

A lies posterior to the inguinal ligament

B must be strangulated if there is no cough impulse over it

C occurs more commonly in a female because of the wider female pelvis

D is invariably acquired, not congenital

E is very liable to strangulate.

23. **The following features are found both in beta cell and non-beta cell islet tumours:**
   A sweating
   B diarrhoea
   C coma
   D abdominal pain
   E the possibility of malignancy.

24. **Pain due to a renal calculus**
   A is not necessarily severe
   B is usually relieved if the patient lies still
   C is often accompanied by vomiting
   D is rarely associated with haematuria
   E is typically intermittent.

25. **A branchial cyst**
   A is a recognized cause of dysphagia
   B can be diagnosed with certainty by microscopical examination of its contents
   C appears at the posterior border of the sternomastoid
   D is embryologically related to a sinus which extends upwards between the internal and external carotid arteries
   E may become infected and rupture externally.

26. **In a patient with a small lax hydrocele, a clue to its aetiology may be provided by**
   A previous prostatectomy
   B a history of mumps in childhood
   C a palpable mass in the abdomen
   D large seminal vesicles palpable on rectal examination
   E nodular thickening of the vas deferens.

## 27. Ulcerative colitis

A  most often affects young males
B  is characterized by abscesses deep in the submucosa
C  may produce a 'drain pipe' colon on barium enema
D  is associated with a specially high risk of malignancy if symptoms start late in life
E  should not be treated with corticosteroids if surgery is likely to be required.


## 28. In the post-operative period

A  the primary treatment of wound infection should be with systemic antibiotics
B  repair of a burst abdomen is usually followed by rapid healing
C  chronic renal failure is associated with poor wound healing
D  50 per cent of deep vein thromboses are undetectable on clinical examination
E  after cholecystectomy retention of stones in the common bile duct is a recognized cause of biliary fistula.


## 29. Deep vein thrombosis

A  is particularly likely to occur in very thin patients
B  in a post-operative patient usually presents clinically within 72 hours
C  can usefully be screened by Doppler ultrasound
D  is best prevented by 5000 units of intravenous heparin twice daily
E  in the femoral veins is more likely to lead to pulmonary embolus than thrombosis in the calf veins.

30. **The following investigations should be carried out routinely in patients presenting with intermittent claudication:**
   A testing for glycosuria
   B haemoglobin
   C electrocardiogram
   D Doppler ultrasound examination of arterial pressure
   E arteriography.

31. **Varicose veins**
   A should be treated by the injection of sclerosing agents only in the elderly
   B are made worse in pregnancy because of hormonal relaxation in smooth muscle
   C recur after surgery only if excision is incomplete
   D may be complicated by phlebitis occurring spontaneously
   E can bleed profusely as a result of minor trauma.

In this section the questions are of the *One-from-Five* type, i.e. only one of the items is correct.

32. **Painful swelling of a submandibular gland is most likely to be due to**
    A  postoperative inflammation
    B  carcinoma
    C  Mikulicz's syndrome
    D  salivary calculus
    E  pleomorphic adenoma.

33. **A patient presents with swelling of all the salivary and the lacrimal glands. The most likely cause is**
    A  tuberculosis
    B  sarcoidosis
    C  Hodgkin's disease
    D  Sjögren's syndrome
    E  lymphosarcoma.

34. **The commonest variety of hernia through the abdominal wall is**
    A  femoral
    B  umbilical
    C  ventral
    D  incisional
    E  inguinal.

35. **The most likely cause of anaemia after partial gastrectomy is**
    A  folate deficiency secondary to steatorrhoea
    B  recurrent haemorrhage from a stomal ulcer
    C  malabsorption of iron
    D  vitamin $B_{12}$ deficiency from loss of intrinsic factor
    E  dietary deficiency of folate due to impaired appetite.

36. **The most common cause of bright red rectal bleeding is**
   A  carcinoma of the rectum
   B  internal haemorrhoids
   C  diverticular disease
   D  fissure-in-ano
   E  ulcerative colitis.

37. **The most common cause of peritonitis is**
   A  perforated peptic ulcer
   B  postoperative leakage from a suture line
   C  septicaemia
   D  acute appendicitis
   E  puerperal infection.

38. **The renal pelvis and calyces are derived from**
   A  the pronephros
   B  the mesonephros
   C  the mesonephric (Wolffian) duct
   D  the metanephros
   E  the metanephric duct.

39. **The best indication that a urinary calculus is made of calcium oxalate is that**
   A  it is sharp and spiky
   B  it is hard and chalky
   C  the urine is infected
   D  it is radio-opaque
   E  it is brown and smooth.

40. **In a patient who has not previously suffered from tuberculosis in any part of the body prostatitis is most likely to be due to**
   A  a virus
   B  a Gram-negative bacillus

C  *M. tuberculosis*
D  a Gram-negative coccus
E  a fungus.

**41. The most common site of malignant disease in the UK is**
A  the large bowel
B  the breast
C  the stomach
D  the uterus
E  none of the above.

**42. Of the following, the most constant feature of primary thyrotoxicosis is**
A  exophthalmos
B  a bruit over the thyroid
C  a rapid pulse
D  diarrhoea
E  atrial fibrillation.

**43. Profuse watery diarrhoea is most likely to be due to**
A  vesico-colic fistula
B  infection with *Clostridium difficile*
C  ulcerative colitis
D  carcinoma of the rectum
E  thyrotoxicosis.

**44. The most common site of a primary carcinoid tumour is the**
A  terminal ileum
B  lung
C  appendix
D  colon
E  liver.

## 45. Both constipation and diarrhoea are recognized features of

**A** uraemia
**B** myxoedema
**C** carcinoma of the colon
**D** fissure-in-ano
**E** Hirschsprung's disease.

The questions in this section are of the *Relationship Analysis* type and you should read the instructions carefully before attempting them.

Each question consists of two statements linked by the word 'because'. The first statement is an assertion and the second an alleged reason for that assertion. The correct answer for each is one of the letters A to E according to the following key:

A  Assertion and reason are true statements and the reason is a correct explanation of the assertion.

B  Assertion and reason are true statements but the reason is not a correct explanation of the assertion.

C  Assertion is true but reason is a false statement.

D  Assertion is false but reason is a true statement.

E  Both assertion and reason are false statements.

46. A cleft lip should be repaired between the 3rd and 6th month *because* the lesion interferes seriously with feeding.

47. The $\beta$-haemolytic streptococcus causes a spreading infection *because* the organism produces enzymes which dissolve the intercellular matrix.

48. Varicocele is commoner on the left than the right *because* renal tumours are commoner on the left.

49. Congenital abnormalities of the diaphragm are common *because* it develops by the fusion of several embryologically distinct structures.

50. Gall bladder disease predisposes to pancreatitis *because* a non-distensible gall bladder allows a rapid rise in biliary pressure with regurgitation along the pancreatic duct.

51. A patient with an insulinoma often puts on a lot of weight *because* the tumour secretes a gastrin-like substance which stimulates the appetite.

52. It is very important to do a biopsy in a suspected case of carcinoma of the pancreas *because* the histological nature of the growth gives a better guide to prognosis than the position of the growth in the gland.

53. Aberrant renal vessels are a common initiating cause of hydronephrosis *because* they frequently cross the dilated renal pelvis at its junction with the ureter.

54. Diverticula of the bladder are commoner in males *because* they are congenital in origin with a sex-linked inheritance.

55. Well-differentiated papillomas of the bladder are more malignant than sessile tumours *because* they form fine fronds, like seaweed, which lead to implantation vesical metastases.

56. It is important to X-ray the chest of patients with urinary retention before embarking on major surgery *because* obstructive renal failure commonly gives rise to an enlarged cardiac silhouette.

57. The prepuce cannot be retracted during the first few months of life *because* there are congenital adhesions between the prepuce and the glans.

**58.** Rupture of the bulbous urethra may present with a suprapubic swelling *because* urine leaks into the extra-peritoneal space.

**59.** Thyroid crisis should be treated by anti-thyroid drugs such as carbimazole *because* these drugs prevent the release of thyroxine from the gland.

**60.** Intestinal obstruction is a common symptom of a Richter's hernia *because* strangulation of the bowel wall frequently occurs.

**61.** Endoscopy should be performed in all cases of bleeding oesophageal varices to establish a diagnosis *because* these patients frequently have peptic ulcers.

# ANSWERS

## PART ONE

| Question | Answer | Question | Answer | Question | Answer |
|---------:|--------|---------:|--------|---------:|-------:|
| 1 | BDE | 26 | ABD | 51 | B |
| 2 | CD | 27 | ABE | 52 | ABCD |
| 3 | AE | 28 | BDE | 53 | BCE |
| *4 | BCD | 29 | ABE | *54 | ABD |
| 5 | ACE | 30 | ABDE | 55 | AB |
| *6 | ACD | 31 | BCE | *56 | AC |
| 7 | BD | 32 | ABCE | 57 | ABCE |
| 8 | ABCE | *33 | BCDE | *58 | AD |
| 9 | B | 34 | ABDE | 59 | ABDE |
| 10 | ADE | 35 | CDE | 60 | ABCDE |
| *11 | D | 36 | ABCDE | 61 | AE |
| *12 | ACD | 37 | ACDE | 62 | BCD |
| 13 | AB | *38 | AE | *63 | ABCD |
| 14 | ABCDE | 39 | ACE | 64 | ADE |
| 15 | BD | 40 | ACD | 65 | AE |
| 16 | ACE | 41 | C | *66 | ABD |
| 17 | ADE | 42 | BCE | *67 | BCE |
| 18 | ACE | *43 | ACE | 68 | AC |
| 19 | CD | 44 | ACDE | 69 | ABDE |
| *20 | BC | 45 | BC | 70 | ABC |
| 21 | ABCE | 46 | AE | 71 | ACDE |
| *22 | ADE | 47 | ACD | 72 | D |
| 23 | ACD | 48 | BCDE | *73 | ABE |
| 24 | ABC | 49 | ABDE | 74 | ABCE |
| *25 | ADE | 50 | ABCE | 75 | BD |

| Question | Answer | Question | Answer | Question | Answer |
|---|---|---|---|---|---|
| 76 | BCD | 102 | C | 128 | BCD |
| 77 | BD | *103 | BD | 129 | BCD |
| 78 | ABDE | 104 | ABD | *130 | All |
| *79 | BC | 105 | DE | | negative |
| 80 | C | *106 | CDE | *131 | BDE |
| 81 | BCE | 107 | BCE | 132 | ADE |
| *82 | ABE | 108 | ABDE | 133 | ABC |
| *83 | ABCE | *109 | AD | 134 | ACE |
| 84 | CDE | 110 | BCE | 135 | BCD |
| 85 | ABD | 111 | ABCD | 136 | ABCD |
| 86 | ABCE | 112 | ACD | *137 | ABCDE |
| *87 | CE | 113 | BC | 138 | ACD |
| 88 | ABCE | 114 | BCDE | 139 | AC |
| 89 | ABDE | *115 | ABDE | 140 | ACDE |
| 90 | BCD | 116 | ABE | 141 | BDE |
| 91 | ACE | 117 | AC | 142 | ACE |
| 92 | ABC | 118 | ABD | *143 | BCE |
| *93 | ABD | 119 | ACE | 144 | ABD |
| 94 | ABD | 120 | BDE | 145 | ABE |
| 95 | AC | 121 | ABE | *146 | BD |
| 96 | BCD | 122 | ABCE | 147 | AC |
| 97 | ACE | *123 | BD | 148 | ACDE |
| 98 | ADE | 124 | BCDE | 149 | B |
| 99 | ABCDE | *125 | A | 150 | CD |
| 100 | CE | 126 | ABC | 151 | ACDE |
| 101 | CE | *127 | BCDE | | |

# ANSWERS

## PART TWO

| Question | Answer | Question | Answer | Question | Answer |
|---|---|---|---|---|---|
| **A** | | **A** | | **C** | |
| 1 | ABE | 26 | ACDE | 46 | C |
| 2 | B | 27 | C | 47 | A |
| 3 | ABCD | 28 | BCDE | 48 | C |
| *4 | ACDE | 29 | CE | 49 | D |
| 5 | CE | 30 | ABCD | 50 | A |
| 6 | BC | 31 | BDE | 51 | C |
| 7 | ABE | | | 52 | E |
| *8 | ACD | | | 53 | D |
| 9 | BDE | | | 54 | C |
| 10 | CDE | **B** | | 55 | E |
| *11 | BCD | *32 | D | 56 | C |
| 12 | ACDE | 33 | B | 57 | A |
| 13 | ABE | *34 | E | 58 | E |
| *14 | DE | 35 | C | 59 | E |
| 15 | CD | *36 | B | 60 | D |
| *16 | AD | *37 | D | 61 | A |
| 17 | ABE | 38 | E | | |
| *18 | ABDE | *39 | A | | |
| *19 | ABCDE | 40 | B | | |
| 20 | ABCD | *41 | E | | |
| *21 | ABCE | *42 | C | | |
| *22 | ACDE | 43 | B | | |
| 23 | BDE | 44 | C | | |
| *24 | AC | 45 | C | | |
| 25 | BDE | | | | |